BACK ABILITY ZERO

BUILD A BETTER BACK WITHOUT LEAVING HOME

Ben, Alissa, Onyx, Sapphire and Lucky Patrick

Copyright © 2023 by Ben Patrick
All rights reserved

This book is printed using paper from registered sustainable and managed sources. No part of this publication may be reproduced, stored in a retrieval system, or transmitted in any form or by any means electronic, mechanical, photocopying, recording or otherwise without the prior permission of the author.

ISBN: 979-8-9851358-3-1

Table of Contents

OPTIONAL WARM-UPS 2

THE BACK ABILITY ZERO WORKOUT 4

ABILITY 13

OPTIONAL WARM-UP #1: 5-MINUTE BACKWARD WALK 16

OPTIONAL WARM-UP #2: 25 TIBIALIS RAISES 19

    STEP 1: ATG SPLIT SQUAT - 30 SECONDS PER SIDE 24

    STEP 2: 25 ATG-STYLE SEATED GOODMORNINGS 28

    STEP 3: 15 PIRIFORMIS PUSH-UPS PER SIDE 32

    STEP 4: 15 SINGLE-LEG PIKES 37

    STEP 5: 15 L-SIT RAISES PER SIDE 41

    STEP 6: 15 QL EXTENSIONS PER SIDE 45

    STEP 7: WALL PULLOVER - 30 SECONDS 49

    STEP 8: 15 TRAP-3 RAISES 51

    STEP 9: COUCH STRETCH - 30 SECONDS PER SIDE 54

CONCLUSION 57

My goal is to provide a full back workout you can use for yourself and others, RIGHT NOW (and forever more), with ZERO gym equipment.

This book features two optional warm-ups and nine exercises that will benefit the back in different ways.

While they could be done daily, I'm a fan of performing them every other day. This leaves extra time for recovery and for other exercises and activities of your choosing.

After going through all the exercises, you could perform a second set on any area you feel you need more work on. The Back Ability sequence is both a workout and a diagnostic tool at the same time.

First up is an overview of the full workout, with an important note for each exercise.

Then I'll break down each exercise individually, showing how to do each as well as the anatomy of how it helps the back. I'll also share the full usage insights I've learned through coaching clients from a broad range of ages and abilities.

I chose to shoot all the photos from home. My wife and I demonstrated while our kids were present so you can see how realistic it is to do this program.

Thank you for giving us a shot.

OPTIONAL WARM-UPS

1. 5 minutes of Backward Walking

I believe this is THE fundamental exercise for foot and knee health. Yes, this is a book about the back, but I've seen the best results when improving abilities from the ground up.

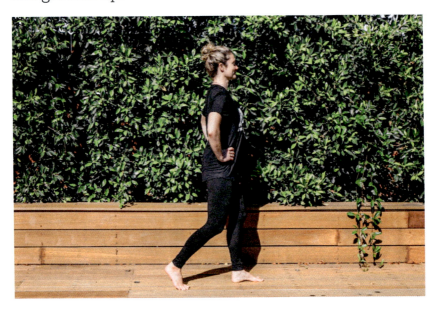

2. 25 Tibialis Raises

You just can't be "too strong" from the ground up. This muscle is chronically underdeveloped, and it's your body's first line of defense against pain and injury. In my opinion, backward walking plus tibialis raises are Mother Nature's opening steps for any exercise program.

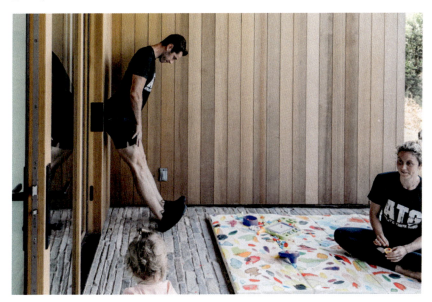

THE BACK ABILITY ZERO WORKOUT

1. ATG (Athletic Truth Group) Split Squat: 30 seconds per side

No single exercise does more to reverse the ill effects of excessive sitting than this one. It improves stiff knees and hips.

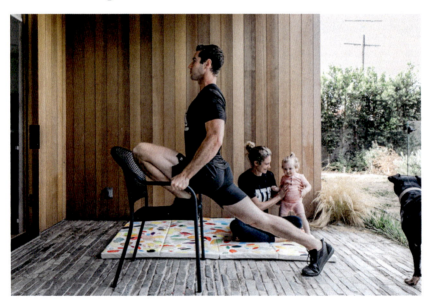

2. Seated Goodmorning: 25 reps

While the ATG Split Squat counters problems due to excessive sitting, we also want to BULLETPROOF that position. The less you deep squat in daily life, the tighter you may be.

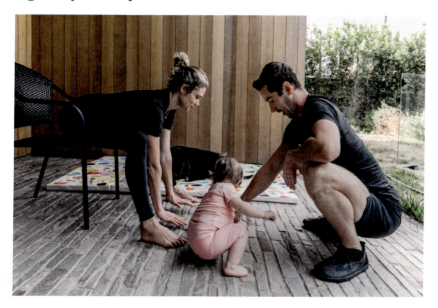

3. Piriformis Push-up: 15 reps per side

As kids we didn't need this, but when we stop sitting and playing like kids, the outer hips can stiffen up, directly leading to restrictions for the back!

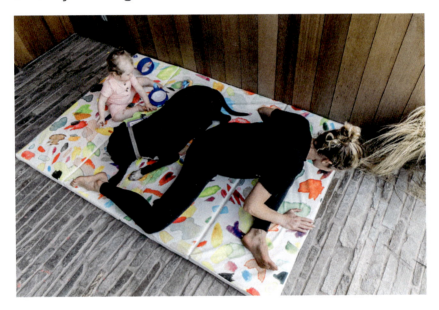

4. Pike Progression: 15 reps per side

Now that we've addressed three tight areas BELOW the back, we get to the back itself, but supported by the hands. Only ABILITY in ALL directions can truly make your back its most protected.

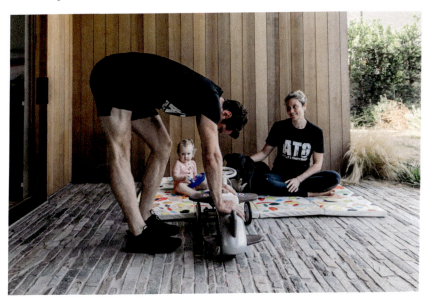

5. L-Sit Progression: 15 reps per side

Time to strengthen the exact opposite of the previous exercise. There is just no escape from ABILITY - and the quest for impressive 6-packs has left society chronically weak BELOW the belly button.

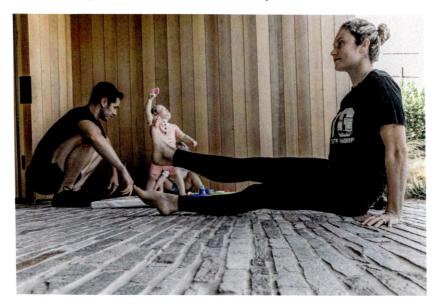

6. QL: 15 reps per side

Rarely trained, this muscle attaches into your lower spine. Strength and flexibility on each side make a more protected spine, because back injuries don't just occur in straight motions!

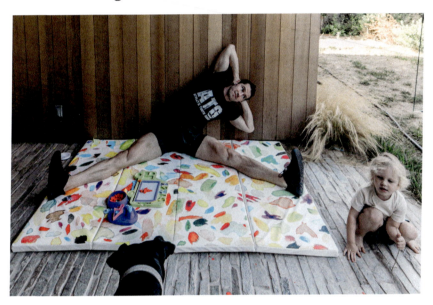

7. Pullover: 15 reps

Now we address what's ABOVE the lower back. Almost all modern backs are too tight in this exercise. It's one of the biggest differences between kids and adults: Ever see a child throw out their back?

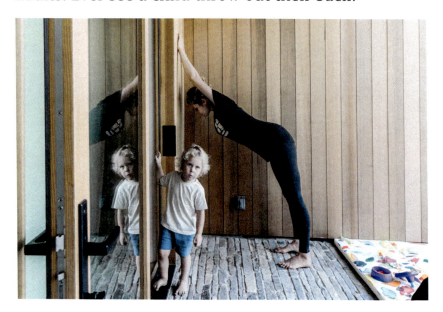

8. Trap-3 Raise: 15 reps

Strength on the opposite side of the last exercise. It may be simple, but it has uncommon progression potential.

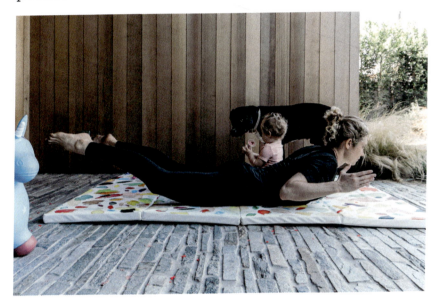

9. Couch Strength: 30 seconds per side

Notice how step 1 and step 9 both stretch the hip flexors? That's intentional. This stretch plus the ATG Split Squat tackle stiff hips and quads in specific ways that make them a consistent one-two punch for long-term transformation.

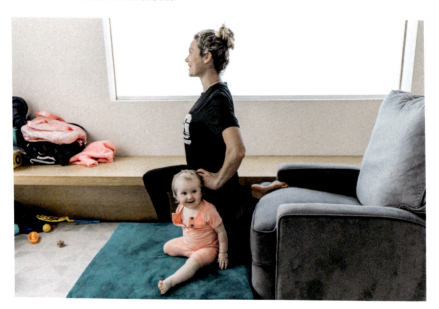

ABILITY

My goal now is to give you a greater understanding of each step listed above so you can use each one to help not only yourself, but anyone in your life who wants more pain-free back ability.

There is one common denominator between all 11 ingredients: ABILITY.

The idea behind "ability training" is that if you have enough ability in the right areas, the body doesn't get hurt and malfunctions eventually vanish!

When a back gets hurt, there must be some degree of force or motion that wasn't easily handled by the body's levels of ability at that time.

Knee Ability Zero offered the first broad education on the following concept, but really it's just common sense: By patiently transforming the ABILITY of my knees, I was able to take the same game that once destroyed my knees - basketball - to a healthy, almost unimaginable level.

Maybe you've seen videos of me jumping off high objects and landing smoothly. I've done such ill-advised demonstrations consistently for years without ever getting hurt.

But let me remind you that it's only a question of ABILITY vs. DEMAND. You'd better believe that if I dropped from high enough, I'd break my legs! The physics of the situation is inescapable.

Therefore, the purpose of this book is not to conjure up a magical reduction of pain, but rather to generate a greater ability to handle life. My goal as your coach is to put the physics more on your side.

Experience has paved routes to SAFELY develop key abilities in relation to the back. These progressions have led to hundreds of success stories from ATG online trainees who achieved a fundamental change in how their backs function, accompanied by chronic pain washing away.

ATG is short for "Athletic Truth Group." I started ATG long before I was KneesOverToesGuy. ATG was a gym for seven years, but eventually demand for its unique system grew beyond our walls. ATG was already short for "ass to grass," which indicates squatting with a full range of motion - thus putting your butt close to the ground. I loved that acronym, so I wanted my gym to fit those letters. I didn't give a whole lot of thought to it at the time, but it's worked out well. If you see me use "ATG" or "ATG-style" before an exercise, it just means we're using a full range of motion in an exercise that isn't commonly done like that.

In many cases the results of the ATG system have seemed "miraculous" - but in *every* case there was an increase of ability relative to the demand of life.

Whatever else someone might do for back pain, whether diet, supplement, or other treatments, ABILITY training is a valuable skill to master.

And so this book is dedicated to all those in the ATG community who have worked with us through these unusual but life-changing exercises.

OPTIONAL WARM-UP #1: 5-MINUTE BACKWARD WALK

Forward walking is a GREAT exercise for longevity.

But when you walk backward, you create additional benefits, starting with strengthening your feet.

There are nearly 30 different muscles associated with the foot and ankle, but in a modern leg, they are largely neglected. Squats, deadlifts, leg presses, leg extensions: These are all legitimate exercises, but the foot doesn't move in any of them. Long-term, this leads to proportionately weak feet compared to the body's intended design.

If you ask me for my go-to solution for foot pain, my answer is backward walking.

Backward walking is how I got myself off painkillers for my knees. It puts your knee in a position where it is under manageable pressure and can get stronger.

"Don't let your knees over your toes" was mainstream advice for decades, simply due to misunderstanding how pressure works. We actually *need* pressure to strengthen the body.

Therefore, the riddle to knee strengthening is solved by UNDERSTANDING knees over toes - not avoiding it or blindly blasting through it without a step-by-step progression.

At the lowest level, you could walk backward in a pool!

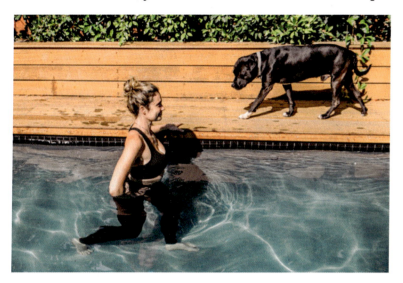

What makes backward walking particularly helpful for the knee is that unlike most strength exercises, it can be made increasingly effective without weights bearing down on you. The smoothest methods of adding resistance are by dragging a sled or using a treadmill with internal resistance.

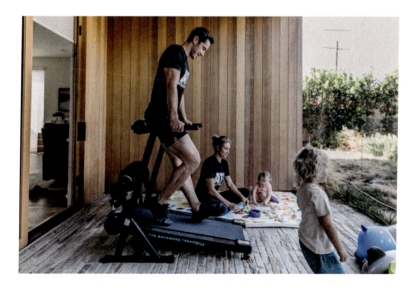

This allows you to improve the ability of your knees with less risk! Even if you increased the resistance to 1,000 pounds, you wouldn't get crushed - the sled or treadmill simply wouldn't move.

The combination of safe ability increases and rhythmic stepping results in improved CIRCULATION to increase healing.

Strength, cardio, healing… all from one exercise! I've never experienced anything quite like it.

Last but not least, backward walking gives you a long-term progression which doesn't aggravate the back. In fact, it's very possible that the increased circulation and abilities can improve the lower back itself.

Before we move on, let's get into three key mental intentions while performing this exercise:

1. Push through your toes.
2. Get into a smooth rhythm.
3. While holding that rhythm, gradually increase the pace!

These simple but important intentions have led people to the most consistent long-term results.

OPTIONAL WARM-UP #2: 25 TIBIALIS RAISES

While backward walking reverses the effects of excessive forward pressure, we can also improve the ability to handle forward pressure!

The first step to doing so is the tibialis raise.

Technically, we're increasing the ability of the "anterior tibialis."

"Anterior" means front, and "tibialis" means "of the tibia." Your tibia is your shinbone.

This muscle starts under the knee and goes all the way down to the inside of your foot.

TIBIALIS

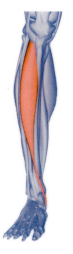
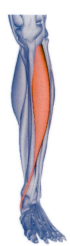

When you walk forward, this is the first muscle that receives the force.

So, even though they're distant from each other, the tibialis helps stabilize the lower back.

With this exercise, we mimic the position in which the tibialis is under load in life, and then we train it as simply as a push-up!

This is like gymnastics for more bulletproofed lower legs:

Lean your butt against a wall. Standing closer to the wall makes it easier, and standing farther makes it tougher.

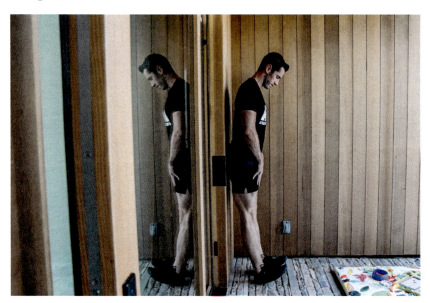

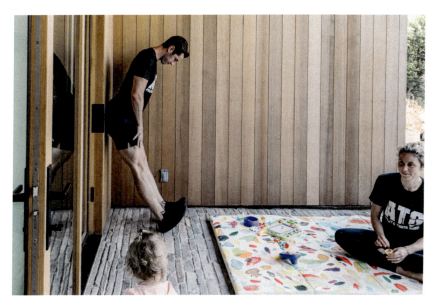

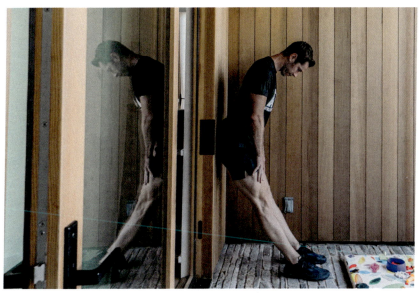

Be sure your back is NOT against the wall, as that actually makes the exercise easier. In coaching thousands through this exercise IN PERSON, I've yet to meet a single one who couldn't achieve an incredible burn. The usual reason someone "doesn't feel it" is that the back is against the wall. That reduces the load of the body, which is what makes this exercise tough.

You should also be aware that I do NOT advise doing this with bare feet on HARD ground. While shoes may not be natural, neither is living on concrete!

As this book continues, we'll get closer and closer to the lower back itself, but I highly encourage you to try each step, no matter how far it might seem to be from your pain.

You never know where your breakthrough might come, and EVERY step of this book - including backward walking and tibialis raises - has been reported as THE solution by some people on the program.

And there's another important reason to train your tibialis:

Let's say you improve the ability of your hips and back to such an extent that you find yourself more active in life: running faster, jumping higher, or just doing your normal activities for longer periods of time without back pain.

Your shins, Achilles, ankles, and feet will now be experiencing greater impacts, and your tibialis helps support these areas.

If a runner dramatically increased knee, hip, and back power, it could manufacture shin pain if the ABILITY of the tibialis didn't increase in logical proportion.

I've come to enjoy these "boring" exercises because they're a constant reminder of how I can now play my sport at full speed without thinking about pain ANYWHERE.

Before we leave tibialis raises, your intention on this exercise is to raise your toes WITHOUT your knees bending. HOLD the top position for a moment. Control the downward movement. PAUSE at the bottom for a moment. Repeat!

STEP 1: ATG SPLIT SQUAT - 30 SECONDS PER SIDE

A stairway offers a perfect regression system.

Elevating the front foot makes the flexibility easier, and assistance from the sides makes the strength easier:

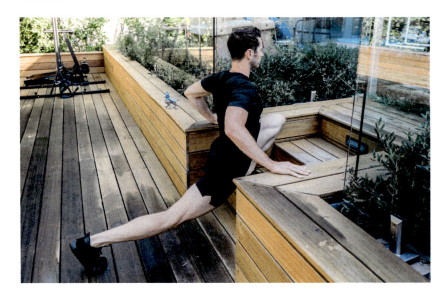

A chair can also work, and then you could find a lower surface to progress.

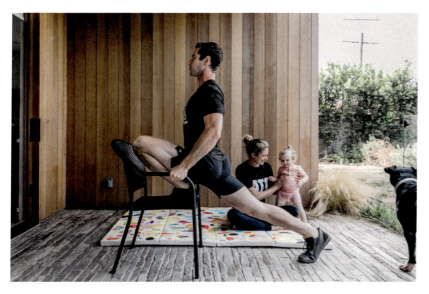

As your ability progresses, you won't need the stairs or chair, other than perhaps for balance, and eventually you won't need that either.

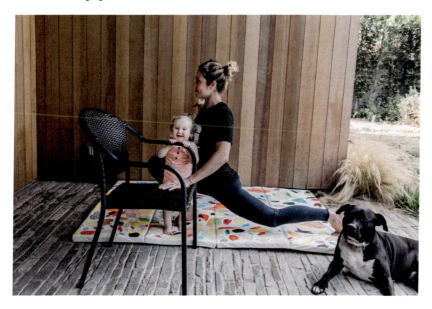

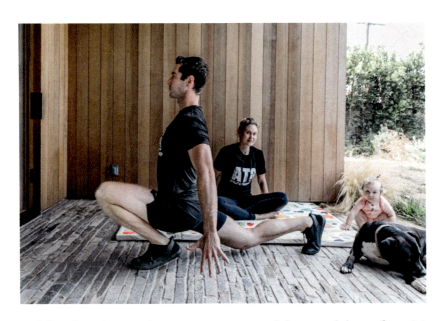

With the intention to master this position for 30 seconds per side, you can create significant changes in the strength *and* length of your hip flexors, a series of five muscles that start from your lower spine and connect all the way to your thigh. They're excessively tight in just about all people, due to a lifestyle of too much sitting:

HIP FLEXORS

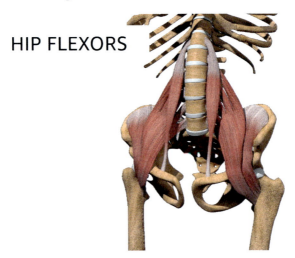

Note: This exercise is a combination of many factors, and there is absolutely nothing wrong with your front heel lifting.

The exercise works regardless of whether your heel is up or down, so find what feels best for you.

STEP 2: 25 ATG-STYLE SEATED GOODMORNINGS

I think of the ATG Split Squat as "reversing" excess sitting, and the seated goodmorning as "bulletproofing" you for excess sitting. I've seen exponential lower back relief when training both of them rather than one or the other.

A chair is perfect to start this exercise. Open your legs wide enough for your torso to sink between them, get your feet in front of your knees, and have the best posture you can.

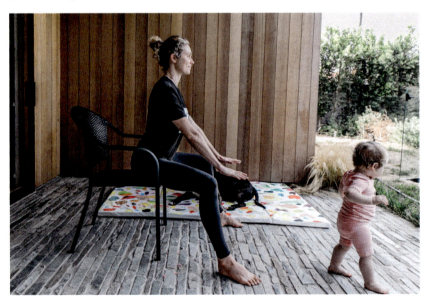

Now reach forward as low as you can without rounding your lower back.

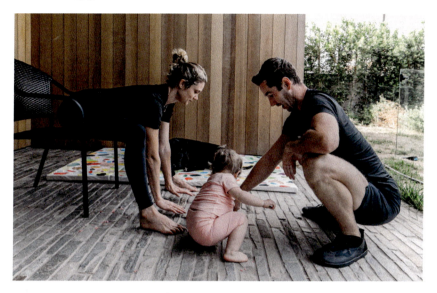

Your goal is to feel a stretch in your adductors, which are your biggest inner thigh muscles.

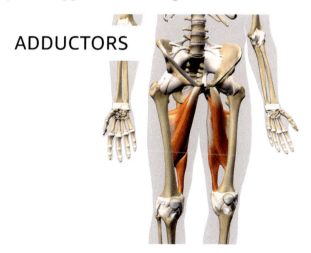

ADDUCTORS

In cultures that stop deep squatting, the inner thighs and hips stiffen up. The seated goodmorning provides a route to get your flexibility more like what it was when you were younger.

There's particular need for patience on this exercise compared to other back exercises:

The stiffer your seated goodmorning, the more your lower back rounds.

Most people have been getting stiffer for years, leaving the lower back in a vulnerable position when squatting or bending over.

By starting with only your bodyweight and putting in the work with high repetitions, we can create new levels of flexibility AND lower back strength!

You have two key intentions on this one:

1. Hold the best posture you can.
2. Reach as deep as you can without rounding your back.

Over time, you could add weight by holding dumbbells in your hands. Through the two intentions above, your flexibility and lower back strength can progress in harmony, eventually leading to a weightlifting bar on your back feeling rock solid in this exercise.

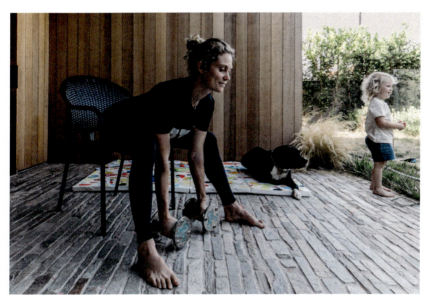

The ATG Split Squat plus ATG-style seated goodmorning have been my favorite combination to help people with the lower back.

If I could teach only these two steps, I would still be very grateful for my job.

STEP 3: 15 PIRIFORMIS PUSH-UPS PER SIDE

The piriformis is a muscle in the outside of your hip. It comes from the words "pear" and "form" because it's shaped like a pear.

Your piriformis is along the path of a nerve that goes from your back down to your legs, so loosening up the piriformis often causes "instant relief" for the lower back. These cases would indicate that patiently working the piriformis to a high level of ability would be part of a well-rounded approach for the lower back.

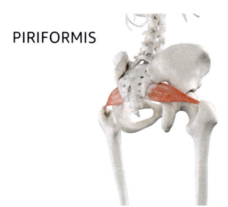

PIRIFORMIS

You may be noticing that "strength-through-length" is a major theme for the lower back. Any area which connects to your lower back and ends up tight OR weak makes your lower back vulnerable!

I believe this is why the lower back is so "mysterious." It's NOT mysterious if you understand all the muscles that connect to it, and have solutions to make them both flexible and strong.

Get in position with your front and back leg each at about 90-degree angles, with your hands on the floor and your front knee in line with your face. If you look closely, little Sapphire is doing this stretch naturally! In fact, I believe that sitting in chairs for so many hours, from such a young age, is one of the reasons our hips tend to get too stiff.

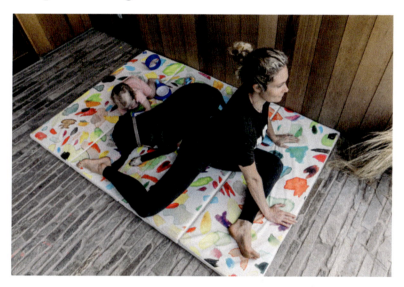

Now, lower your chest until you feel a stretch:

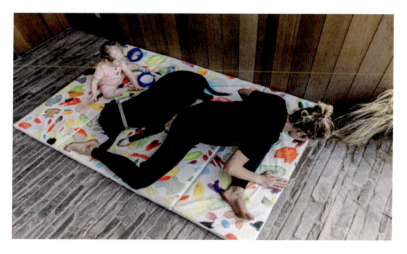

Then, push back up to the starting position, using your hands AND the strength of your outer hip muscles, by thinking about pushing your front knee into the floor.

When this feels easy, remove your inside hand so you have even more load on the piriformis.

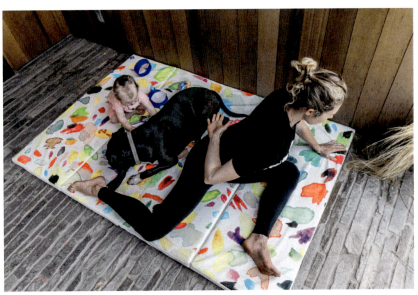

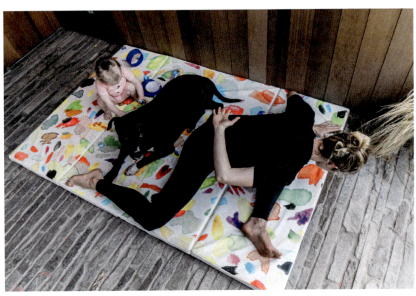

Early on, you might not be able to get into the starting position comfortably. If so, put a pillow or pad under the outside hip, like this:

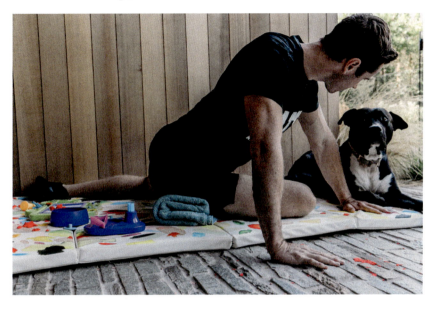

Now is a good time to remind you that from person to person, you'll often find significant variance in ability from exercise to exercise. That's why I like to go through all of them, then return to your particular tight (or weak) spots for a second round.

Your intention on this exercise is to get into a stretched position in your outer hip, and then use the strength of the outer hip to push yourself back up with as little assistance from the hands as possible.

Of course, there is NO RUSH. I want you to get some enjoyment from these motions. Improving strength and flexibility is work, but it definitely shouldn't be painful.

For example, it would be better to use a smaller amount of motion than it would be to wince your way through a stretch that you can't control.

Over the course of workouts - a week, a month, a year - I believe you CAN re-engineer the protection of your lower back, but working through pain doesn't seem to speed your progress.

You may notice that Steps 1 through 3 address commonly stiff areas BELOW the lower back:

1. The hip flexors
2. The adductors
3. The piriformis

I think of these as the "Below The Lower Back" segment of Back Ability.

The next three steps I think of as "AROUND The Lower Back."

STEP 4: 15 SINGLE-LEG PIKES

Now we're seeking the gentlest way to address the lower back's ability to BE in a rounded position.

Steps 1-3 are all about preventing stress on the lower back. Step 4 is about being able to TOLERATE that stress.

This exercise improves both the strength and flexibility needed to be in a rounded position.

Higher support for the hands makes it easier. Lower makes it tougher.

Start with bent knees.

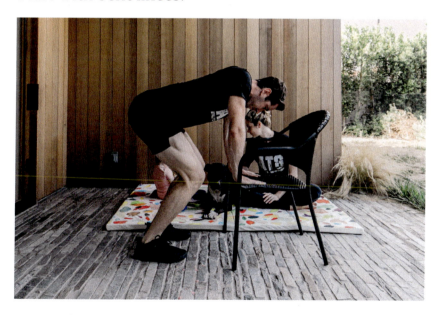

Then straighten one leg.

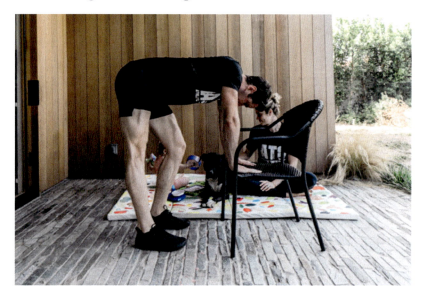

Return to the bent knee position. Then repeat with the other leg.

Perform 15 reps per side.

If the stretch is easy, go lower:

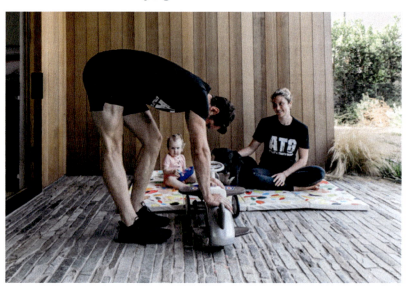

One of the goals of Back Ability is palms to floor while doing this exercise:

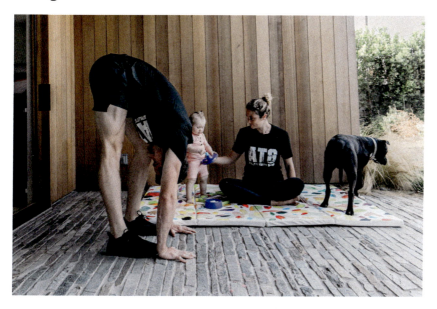

Since your hands support your body's weight, you can spend time stimulating your spine in a rounded position, without excess stress. The goal is being comfortable and capable in that position.

There is no one magic movement for the lower back.

This is one ability of the back. There are many others. Your best chances in life will come from ability in all of them.

A rounded back got a bad reputation despite lack of evidence. But it's understandable why: It appears to be a more vulnerable position, and that might be true.

But just because a position is vulnerable, that doesn't mean we should run away from ability in that area. For many people, improvement on this exercise has resulted in greater freedom and less pain for the lower back.

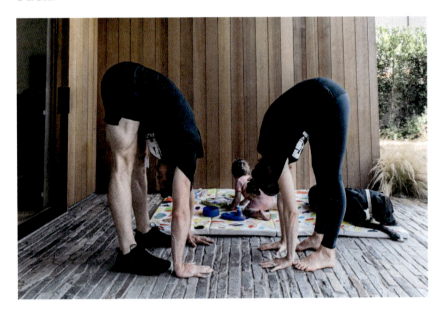

STEP 5: 15 L-SIT RAISES PER SIDE

This strengthens the opposing muscles of the previous exercise! A body with ability on both sides is more bulletproof than one with ability on one side but not the other.

Two excellent goals in the ATG exercise system are the palms to floor pike and the L-sit with body fully off the floor. But most people need to start this exercise at a lower level...

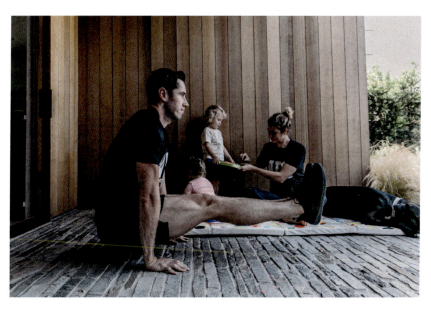

Sit on the floor, with legs straight. Feel your hip flexor work to lift your leg. Hold 2 seconds. Lower. Repeat with the other leg. Perform 15 reps per side.

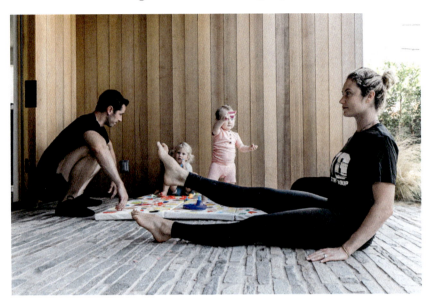

Leaning back makes it easier:

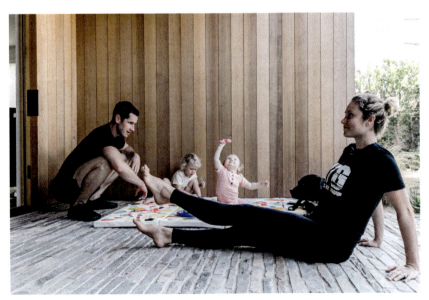

And having a leg *plus* your glutes off the ground makes it tougher!

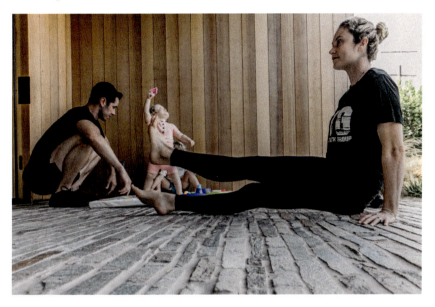

The L-sit trains the strength of the hip flexors while also developing deep core muscles.

I believe this gives the lower back greater stability, even though hip flexor strength has often been discouraged because you "don't want to stiffen up."

But strengthening a muscle doesn't inherently make it stiffer.

A better solution is creating flexible AND strong hip flexors. Thanks to the ATG Split Squat as the foundation, you can absolutely improve both qualities simultaneously.

Your intention on this exercise is to exhaust those hip flexor muscles, but at a level that doesn't cause excess strain. By exhausting them, recovering, and repeating, you can consistently build hip flexor strength above the norm.

STEP 6: 15 QL EXTENSIONS PER SIDE

QL is short for *quadratus lumborum*. Think "quad" because of its four sections. Look closely at the picture below and you'll see how each one attaches into the lower spine! "Lumborum" means "of the lumbar spine" and "lumbar" is the name of the lower back's portion of your spine.

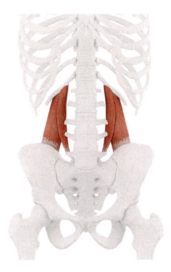

QUADRATUS LUMBORUM

When interviewing people with back injuries, it quickly becomes apparent that a good percentage of these injuries happen with LATERAL forces involved, not just straight forward and backward pressures. You bend down to pick up something that isn't directly in front of you and... BOOM! Now you're relying on your QL muscle!

The QL is rarely ever trained with strength-through-length, so start slow because it can make you quite sore. Many people who've been exercising for decades never trained this muscle, so it's like being a newbie all over again. But I think of it like this: new muscle, new potential!

Sitting with your back against a wall and legs spread apart for stability, stretch your body to one side until you feel the QL stretch. Go back and forth 15 times per side. The leverage of your arms makes the exercise either easier or harder.

Easier:

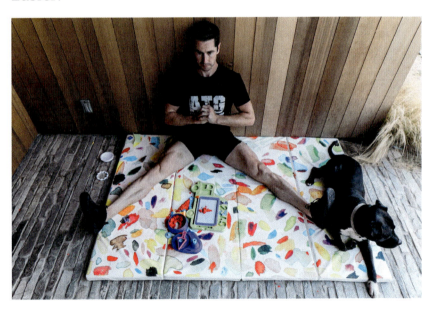

Harder:

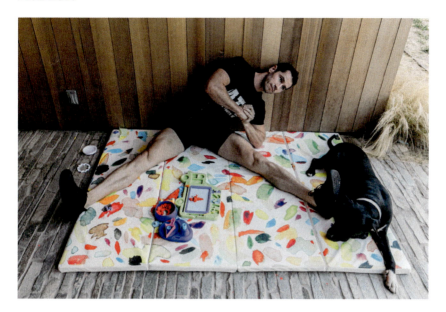

Even Harder:

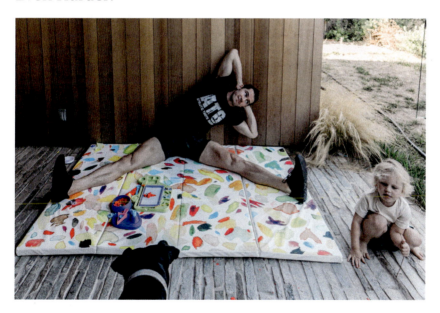

Hardest:

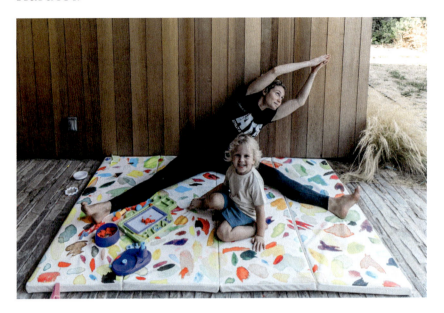

Adding the QL to the previous two exercises now gives us ability all around the lower spine.

STEP 7: WALL PULLOVER - 30 SECONDS

Now we address strength and mobility ABOVE your lower back.

A wall is a great place to begin this step.

With hands together and overhead, walk your feet back until you feel a gentle stretch through your upper body.

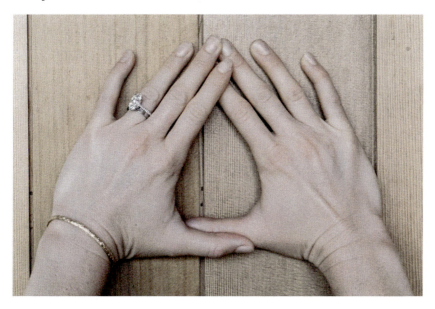

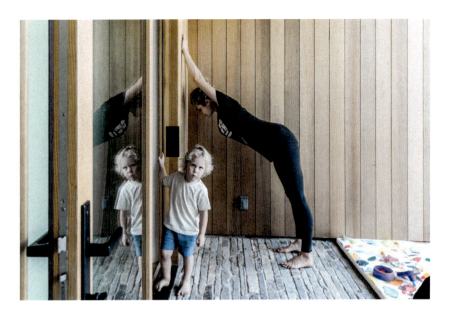

Your goal is to feel *strong* in this position.

This opens up your posture in the opposite direction of the modern hunch while increasing upper body strength through a variety of muscles in your arms, chest, and back.

This might be the most needed upper body category because the more your upper back stiffens, the more your lower back becomes the breaking point of your body.

STEP 8: 15 TRAP-3 RAISES

The "trap-3" is your third and lowest row of trap muscles (think trapezoid due to their shape).

This third row is JUST above your lower back. It's chronically weak in modern society, likely due to how much time we spend sitting and looking down.

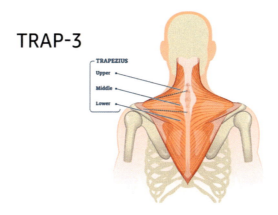

The easiest way to start this is face down on the floor.

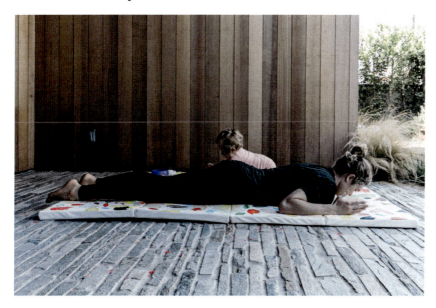

With arms bent, raise your shoulders and legs off the ground.

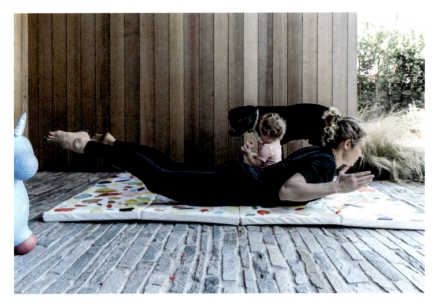

Then extend your arms.

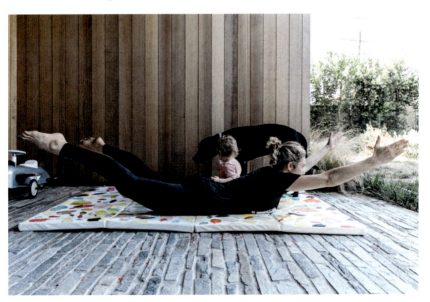

Then slowly lower down.

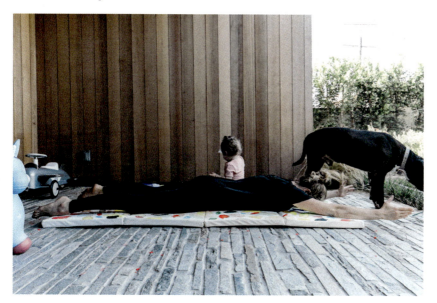

Do this 15 times, at your own pace. You can take breaks as needed.

Then there's one thing that finishes off this workout perfectly...

STEP 9: COUCH STRETCH - 30 SECONDS PER SIDE

I've seen exponential hip flexibility results when using both the ATG Split Squat and the couch stretch, rather than one or the other.

While the ATG Split Squat may allow more gains for the upper portion of your hip flexors which attach into your spine, the couch stretch allows a greater stretch of the lower portion of your hip flexors which attach down into your thigh.

The lowest of the hip flexor muscles is called the *rectus femoris* (*rectus* "straighten" and *femoris* "of the thigh bone"). The rectus femoris happens to work as both a hip flexor and a knee extensor, meaning it extends (straightens) your knee. This may help explain why the couch stretch so commonly gives results for both the knees and the lower back.

RECTUS FEMORIS

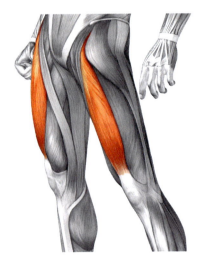

A real couch is great to start with because you can use a soft couch cushion to get into position comfortably:

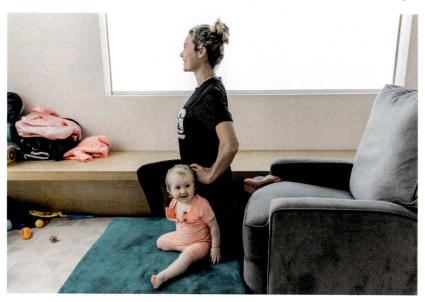

Using a wall is tougher than using a couch, due to the reduced angle of your shin to your thigh. Use what feels best for you.

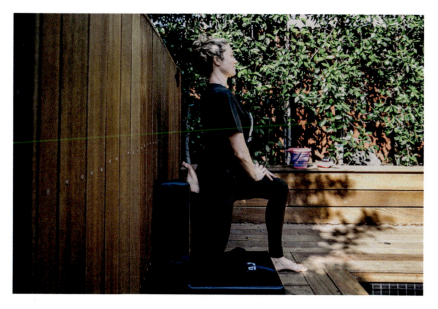

Once in position, I want you to think about two things. I've observed that these lead to greater long-term gains:

1. Squeeze the glute (butt) muscle of the side you're stretching. You'll immediately notice how this increases the stretch for your hip flexors.

2. Think as if you're gently kicking into the couch or mat. Over time, this allows you to make your rectus femoris stronger in its stretched position.

CONCLUSION

Thank you for using this book.

I believe strongly that pursuing ABILITY will give you much greater long-term outcomes than avoidance will.

Some of the methods in this book are still unconventional, so I appreciate your willingness to learn them.

While you may have found me on social media, I built my career on in-person results. When in-person demand exceeded what I could handle, I put my system online.

At ATGonlinecoaching.com, you get full access to all ATG programs, and we answer your questions and coach your videos in less than 24 hours, 7 days a week, with no monthly contract.

We also work to make the ATG system more comfortable and accessible through equipment such as our Backward Treadmill, all available at ATGequipment.com.

Through whatever combination of reading, coaching and equipment works best for you, I hope you gain tools to help yourself and others for the rest of your life.

Yours in Solutions,

Ben

Made in the USA
Las Vegas, NV
28 February 2024

86377364R00038